LET'S TALK ABOUT... SEXUAL FANTASIES AND DESIRES

Questions and Conversation Starters for Couples Exploring Their Sexual Interests

What turns *you* on?

J.R. James

Beyond the Sheets Series

Book 1

ISBN: 9781796993196

Spice up your sex life even more, and explore all the *Let's Talk About...* sexy discussion books by J.R. James:

Let's Talk Sexy
All **THREE** *Let's Talk About...* sexy question books in one massive volume for one low price. Save now!

Let's Talk About... Sexual Fantasies and Desires
Recharge your passion as you delve into sexual fantasies and examine your sexual interests. Explore your partner's sexual past and discover what really arouses them. The erotic energy is cranked up as you uncover things never revealed and express your true sexual turn-ons!

Let's Talk About... Non-Monogamy
Interested in Open Relationships, Swinging, or Polyamory? If you're exploring or already enjoying ethical non-monogamy of any kind, these revealing conversational questions will help you and your partner mutually examine and discuss sexual desires, boundaries, and expectations.

Let's Talk About... Kinks and Fetishes
Are you looking to expand sexual horizons with your lover? Do you want to get freaky in the bedroom, but don't know where to start? If you've got an inner wild child just aching to get out, then this book is for you.

DEDICATION

To RJ,
The sexiest woman I know and my best friend. May our lives be filled with many more adventures and laughs.

Sign up for our mailing list and be entered to win a **FREE** copy of any of the *Let's Talk About...* sexy question books. New winner selected every month!

Sign up here:

https://mailchi.mp/a75ed05fd334/jrjames

What This Book is About

Several summers ago, my wife and I were on a cross-country trip. As we drove through the rolling hills and golden plains of the Midwest, we did all the normal things a couple might do on a road trip together. We talked, listened to music, and played random silly games to pass the time. In preparation for our long drive, I had bought a "question book" for couples. As we took turns at the wheel, we had fun asking each other the light hearted questions the book offered.

On one of the pages, there were a few sexy "Would you consider..." type questions. My wife was the one driving, so it was my turn to do the asking. As I read the page, my heart skipped a beat. One of the questions was a huge sexual fantasy of mine. For whatever reason, it was something I had never felt comfortable sharing with her, but here was my chance to actually ask her what she thought about it. The best part? It wasn't really *me* asking the question, it was the *book!* I'll never forget the electric thrill I experienced when she rolled the question over in her mind for a moment then answered, "Yeah, I might be open to that."

That answer kicked off what I consider to be the hottest, most erotic conversation of my life. We had been together approximately eight years, and yet, it felt like I was rediscovering her sexual presence for the first time. That afternoon in the car will forever be with me, and my pulse still quickens when I think of it. This one sexually charged conversation led to many amazing adventures and discussions in the years that have followed.

The experience gave me pause as I realized that we often "hold back" our secret fantasies, desires, or passions from our partner without even knowing it. Whether from shame or embarrassment, intentionally or unintentionally, people may never share what *really turns them on*. That's what this book is meant to do. It is a tool that enables you to ask questions and explore your partner's likes, dislikes, desires, and fantasies.

It doesn't matter whether you've been dating a week or married ten years, whether you're straight, bi, gay, lesbian, or other, there are questions in here for everyone. The conversation starters in this book vary from mild to explicit. If you're uncomfortable with a specific question, move on to another. Some of the couples reading this book may think they already know everything there is to know about their partner. I still recommend going through all the questions. Your partner may just surprise you.

Whether you read this surrounded by candles and sipping a glass of wine, or during a long road trip, or even at a party with other couples, keep your ears, hearts, and minds open. Be understanding. Be honest. And remember, discussion is key.

Enjoy!

What This Book is Not

This book is meant to push boundaries. That being said, it is not intended for insecure couples or individuals, or those who might be prone to jealousy.

This book is not intended to replace therapeutic discussion and is for entertainment purposes only. If you and a partner have sexual or relational problems, we strongly recommend seeing a sex or marriage therapist.

We are not recommending any of the things in this book, nor do we encourage any actions or behaviors outside of a person's comfort limits. In addition, we do not encourage or recommend any unsafe sex practices.

The conversation starters in this book are not meant to be a comprehensive list of every fetish, kink, or fantasy. They are simply starters that will, hopefully, lead you into deeper discussions. So please, feel free to elaborate and improvise on the questions. ;)

1

What are the favorite areas of your body you like to be kissed? Any unusual erogenous zones?

2

Besides the bedroom, where else in your home would you like to have sex?

3

Describe one fantasy you've never shared with anyone else.

4

Outside of your home, where is one place you'd like to have sex?

5

Name one famous person you'd like to spend a night of passion with. What's sexy about that person?

6

What do you think about role playing or dressing up? Describe a role playing scenario that would turn you on.

7

Do you like using toys in the bedroom? What are your favorites? Are there any you don't have that you'd like to try?

8

How would you feel about watching your partner make out with another person? How about watching them have sex?

9

Describe from start to finish your idea of an erotic date.

10

Name three songs you'd like to listen to while having sex. Why those songs?

11

Tell your partner what their most attractive physical attributes are.

12

What's sexier, a hot body, hilarious personality, or a brilliant mind?

13

If someone had to watch you and your partner have sex, who would it be?

14

Name two foods you consider sexy or that you would like to use during sex.

15

What are some of the sexiest items of clothing your partner wears? Is there anything else you'd like to see them in?

16

Is there a sexual position you've always wanted to try, but never have?

17

Do you like to talk dirty or hear your lover talk dirty? If so, what kind of things do you like to say or hear?

18

What is your favorite sexual position? Why?

19

Have you ever played strip poker (or any other strip game)? If so, describe what happened. If not, would you consider it?

20

Have you ever gone skinny dipping? If so, was it an erotic experience? If not, would you consider it?

21

Would you ever consider swinging or swapping partners? If so, are there any friends you could imagine joining you and your partner in the bedroom?

22

How would you feel about having sex "secretly" with your partner with other people nearby?

23

Excluding pornography, are there any movies that turn you on? Why?

24

What kind of mood lighting do you find sexy?

25

If you were a porn star, what would your first movie be titled, and what would it be about?

26

Is it a turn on to see your partner flirt with others?

27

Have you ever had sex in a public place? If not, would you consider it? Where would it be?

28

Have you ever had sex at work? If not, would you? Where and how would you do it?

29

What is the sexiest dream you've ever had?

30

Do you like to dominate or be submissive?

31

Would you ever consider participating in an amateur striptease? What songs would you dance to?

32

Describe your first sexual experience. Is there anything about it you would have changed?

33

Have you ever fantasized about being forced to watch your partner pleasure someone else?

34

Have you ever had a one night stand? If so, describe what happened?

35

Have you ever been caught masturbating? If so, by whom? What did you do when you were caught?

36

Would you ever consider participating in an orgy? If so, what would be the prerequisites?

37

Would you ever try a nude beach or a clothing-optional resort?

38

Which parts of a woman's body are the most sexually attractive?

39

Which parts of a man's body is the most sexually attractive?

40

Would you prefer to see your partner fool around with a member of the same sex or of the opposite sex?

41

What turns you on the most during sex?

42

What do you like to do after sex?

43

What do you like to see a woman wear to bed? What do you like to see a man wear?

44

*Have you ever had
something embarrassing
happen during sex?*

45

Are you loud or quiet in bed? Do you like to hear your partner's enjoyment?

46

When was the last time you masturbated? What were you thinking about?

47

What is your understanding of "non-monogamy" and what do you think about it?

48

What kinks or fetishes do you have an interest in?

49

Are there any kinks or fetishes you've already tried?

50

What do you know about tantric sex? Have you ever tried it?

51

Would you consider having sex in front of other people while they watched?

52

Would you like to watch another couple have sex in the same room as you?

53

Have you ever been to any sort of sex class? If not, what is a class you would like to experience?

54

What is the thing you do best in bed? How did you get so good at it?

55

What kind of kissing do you like best? Current partner excluded, who was the best kisser you've ever experienced?

56

How do you like to flirt,
and how do you like others
to flirt with you?

57

How do you like your partner to initiate sex? What's your favorite way of initiating?

58

Lights on or lights off?
Why?

59

What's the sexiest "non-sexual" thing someone can do to turn you on?

60

Has anyone ever taken sexy photos of you? Have you ever taken any of someone else?

61

Out of all your past sexual partners (present partner excluded), who was the best and why?

62

Do you find uniforms sexy? If so, what kind?

63

Can jealousy ever feel erotic? Try and describe why you think it can or can't be.

64

Have you ever had sex in a car? If not, would you try it?

65

How many times a week is the ideal amount to have sex?

66

Is there a specific orgasm you've had in your life that particularly stands out?

67

Are massages ever arousing? Have you ever had an "innocent" massage lead to sex?

68

Which do you prefer for the pubic area, hair or no hair?

69

*Have you ever tried anal
sex? If so, how was it?
Any anal play fantasies?*

70

Does size matter? Why or why not?

71

Have you ever tried handcuffs or bondage? If not, would you like to?

72

Which is more erotic, being blindfolded yourself or blindfolding your partner?

73

Have you ever received, or have ever given, a lap dance?

74

*What is your favorite time
of day to have sex?*

75

What part of your body are you most proud of?

76

Is there anything you'd enjoy watching me do either solo or with another person?

77

What helps you relax so that you can be fully present during sex?

78

Finish this sentence: I always love it when you…

79

If you had the chance to sleep with one person besides me, who would it be?

80

Who's the most "inappropriate" person you've ever fantasized about?

81

If you had to choose one person, we both know, for me to sleep with one time, who would it be and why?

82

How many sexual partners have you had in the past? Does oral sex count?

83

Have you ever had sex with a stranger? If not, how much money would it take to have sex with an attractive stranger? With an "average" stranger?

84

Have you ever faked an orgasm? If so, why? Give a demonstration of faking an orgasm.

85

What's the least amount of time you've known someone before sleeping with them?

86

What's the shortest amount of time that has elapsed between having sex with two different partners?

87

Can you recall a particular sexual encounter that lasted an unusually long time? Describe the encounter.

88

Have you ever been attracted to a friend's mother or father? If so, describe them.

89

Have you ever thought about someone else other than your lover during sex?

90

What do you think about porn? If you were watching a porn video, describe a scene that would arouse you.

91

Have you ever had phone sex? If not, would you? What kind of things would you say?

92

How do you feel about sexting? What's the sexiest thing you can text someone?

93

Where's the strangest place you've ever masturbated? Is there anywhere else you'd be willing to try?

94

What do you know about the book of Kama Sutra? Have you ever tried anything from it?

95

Have you ever fantasized about one of your teachers? If so, describe them. If the chance had presented itself, would you have slept with them?

96

How do you feel about "hall passes"? (Temporary permission to sleep with someone else.)

97

Which leads to hotter sex,
romance or straight up
erotic energy?

98

Have you ever had a threesome? If not, would you consider it? Would you prefer your third to be a man or a woman?

99

If applicable, where do you like to ejaculate or to receive your partner's ejaculate?

100

Is there anything you consider completely "off-limits"? Why? Is there anything that could ever change your mind?

101

Do you prefer your sex gentle or rough?

102

Have you ever secretly masturbated with other people around?

103

Do you like to pull hair or have your hair pulled during sex?

104

Do you like to spank or be spanked?

105

What do you think about BDSM? Is there anything you'd be willing to try if you haven't already?

106

Is foreplay overrated or underrated? Describe your idea of hot foreplay.

107

What's one thing you should absolutely know how to do well to turn me on?

Thank you for reading! Hopefully, these conversations have benefited you and your partner. If you've enjoyed this book, please leave a gracious review on Amazon.

Spice up your sex life even more, and explore all the *Let's Talk About...* sexy discussion books by J.R. James:

Let's Talk Sexy
All **THREE** *Let's Talk About...* sexy question books in one massive volume for one low price. Save now!

Let's Talk About... Sexual Fantasies and Desires
Recharge your passion as you delve into sexual fantasies and examine your sexual interests. Explore your partner's sexual past and discover what really arouses them. The erotic energy is cranked up as you uncover things never revealed and express your true sexual turn-ons!

Let's Talk About... Non-Monogamy
Interested in Open Relationships,
Swinging, or Polyamory? If you're
exploring or already enjoying ethical non-
monogamy of any kind, these revealing
conversational questions will help you and
your partner mutually examine and
discuss sexual desires, boundaries, and
expectations.

Let's Talk About... Kinks and Fetishes
Are you looking to expand sexual horizons
with your lover? Do you want to get freaky
in the bedroom, but don't know where to
start? If you've got an inner wild child just
aching to get out, then this book is for you.

Made in the USA
San Bernardino, CA
11 February 2020

64370876R00073